God's
Good Gift

God's Good Gift

Teaching Your
Kids About Sex
– Ages 8 to 11

Mary Ann Mayo

ZondervanPublishingHouse
Grand Rapids, Michigan

A Division of HarperCollinsPublishers

If you are interested in having them come to your community for a seminar on communicating with children about sex:

DECENT DISCLOSURE
HOW TO RAISE MORALLY RESPONSIBLE CHILDREN
IN AN IRRESPONSIBLE WORLD

Dr. and Mrs. Mayo may be contacted by writing to:
Reference Point, Box 8022, Redlands, California, 92375

GOD'S GOOD GIFT
Teaching Your Kids About Sex—Ages 8 to 11
Copyright © 1991 by Mary Ann Mayo

Requests for information should be addressed to:
Zondervan Publishing House
1415 Lake Drive, S.E.
Grand Rapids, Michigan 49506

Library of Congress Cataloging-in-Publication Data

Mayo, Mary Ann.
    God's good gift : teaching your kids about sex : ages 8 to 11 /
Mary Ann Mayo : illustrated by Miriam Wingerd.
      p. cm.
    Summary: Uses a Christian perspective to provide sex instruction
in the context of the family.
    ISBN 0-310-53470-4 (acid-free paper)
    1. Sex instruction. 2. Sex instruction—Religious aspects—
Christianity. [1. Sex instruction for children. 2. Christian
life.] I. Wingerd, Miriam. II. Title.
HQ53.M414   1991
649'.65—dc20
                                   90–26709
                                      CIP
                                      AC

All Scripture quotations, unless otherwise noted, are taken from the *Holy Bible: New International Version* (North American Edition). Copyright © 1973, 1978, 1984 by the International Bible Society. Used by permission of Zondervan Bible Publishers.

Edited by Mary McCormick
Designed by Rachel Hostetter
Illustrated by Miriam Wingerd

Printed in the United States of America

91 92 93 94 95 / AK / 10 9 8 7 6 5 4 3 2 1

This edition is printed on acid-free paper and meets the American National Standards Institute Z39.48 standard.

*This book is dedicated to our husbands, Dan and Joe,
without whom we wouldn't know what a
blessing a family can be!*

*We love you
—Miriam and Mary Ann*

A Note to Parents

Yes, this is another book about sex. A quick look, however, will reveal that it is different from most other books on the subject. Gone are the graphic details straight out of *Gray's Anatomy*. Missing also is a focus on the facts. The emphasis of *God's Good Gift* is to place sexuality into its correct and most meaningful context ... the *family*.

Sex was not created to be the one-dimensional physical release that so much of the media suggests it is. Yes, it's pleasurable; yes, it's exciting ... but there is *more*. Sex finds its greatest meaning, significance, and pleasure within the context of *marital* relationship.

Much of this book presents God's plan for His *gift* of sex. But some segments look at what happens when we misuse, misunderstand, or misinterpret the gift. The truth is that our best is achieved when we determine to live life in a manner that acknowledges the Designer's intent.

Chances are you have struggled with sexual choices. If your family or situation does not match the "ideal," I hope that you will find the text sensitive. My prayer is that you will be able to use the book not only as a tool to reinforce God's best for your child but also to encourage communication and insight into your particular circumstance.

Perhaps some of you worry that children ages eight to eleven need not be exposed to topics such as AIDS, or pornography, or molestation. In reality, it is probable that we are off by five years in our estimation of what our children should know. Recently, a friend's child was unable to sleep. When asked what was bothering him, he confessed that he feared he had contracted AIDS, because a younger child "who had a big head and was real skinny" had spit on him. Our children deserve to know the facts about vitally important matters that affect them.

One can hardly pick up the newspaper without noting another incident of molestation, abduction, or rape of children. We cannot absolve ourselves of our responsibility to provide protection from those who have not been exposed to healthy sex education. Some of you grasp firsthand the lifelong repercussions of not knowing how to protect yourself, or even that you **can** protect yourself.

Frequently, such "truth" is taught to the exclusion of another truth ... that sex is a *gift* and was meant to be good. It is designed for pleasure, for bonding, to assuage loneliness, and for reproduction.

God's Good Gift seeks to correct the imbalance by emphasizing that God has designed our sexuality with meaning and purpose—that each gender contributes to the enrichment of the other—that males and females bring more to one another than physically different bodies—that their sexual design is molded from God's own clay. Because God is certainly not embarrassed that we are sexual creatures, neither should we be.

Although the text clearly emphasizes the broader scope of a person's sexuality, the fact that sexuality is intimately related to the creation of new life is worthy of special attention, especially in a world that devalues "nonproductive" human life.

Miriam Wingerd's beautiful art contributes to this broader appreciation of sexuality by capturing the feeling and essence of the impact of sexuality on human beings (as, for example, in the admiring family around the new baby).

Read this book to your children. Leave it around for them to pick up on their own. Reread it. Talk some more. Keep the lines of communication open. No matter whether your school does a poor or good job of sex education, **you** are and will remain the most influential teacher of sexuality for your children.

May this book be a valuable tool for you and them.

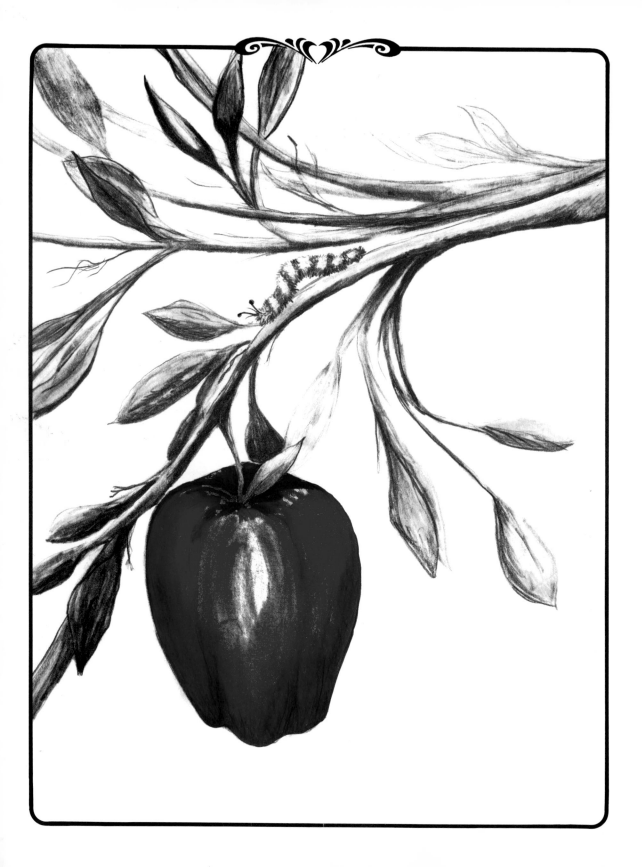

In the beginning, God created the heavens and the earth. Imagine how quiet it would be if he had stopped there! And how boring—if there were no birds swooping through the air majestically balanced on the winds .... no lion creeping slowly and steadily upon an unsuspecting prey ... no caterpillar squinching its way along a branch to a juicy red apple!

Imagine the earth without people!—without kids dodging and darting the keep-away ball—without laughter and screams on the playground, or without kids cheering their team on at school games!

What if there were never a soft lullaby melodiously drifting through a window as a mother comforts her newborn ... or never a family around the dinner table sharing the events of the day?

Aren't you glad that God's plan included plants, animals— and people, too?

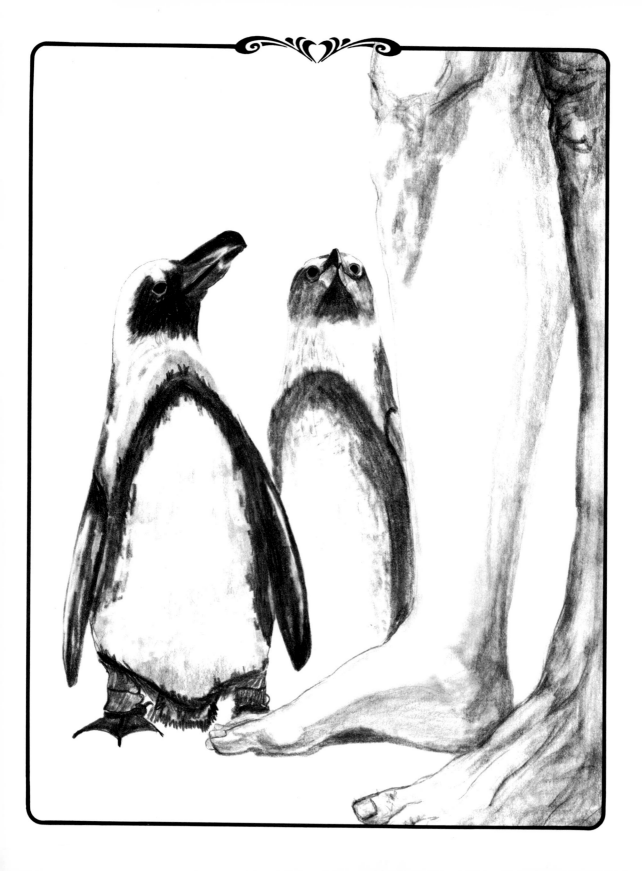

The very first person created was Adam. It didn't take Adam long to realize that something didn't seem quite right. Although the animals had been made in two kinds—male and female—he was all alone.

But God knew that Adam was lonely.

Adam didn't know that God intended to make two kinds of humans—male and also female. To make a perfect match, God used the same material He had used to make Adam, and He formed Eve.

As made-for-each-other companions, men and women were to work and play together. They were designed to depend upon and need each other. They were to be *partners* in taking care of the earth. Most important, unlike the animals, they were made to know who God is and to be His friend.

Adam and Eve were the very first family.

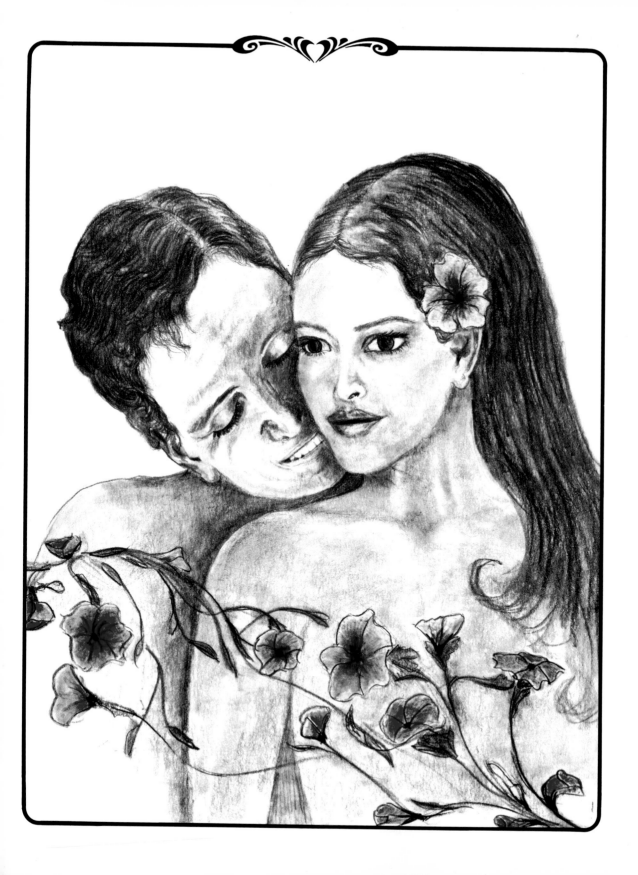

From the very beginning, God decided that when boys and girls grow up and fall in love, they should leave their mothers and fathers begin their own families.

God designed the family to protect children and help them grow up safely. Because He wants each child to have a mother and a father, God made it impossible for a woman to have a baby all by herself or for a man to have a baby all by himself.

No one should be embarrassed because a male and female are necessary for a baby to be created, because the two different kinds of bodies—two sexes—were God's idea.

Babies begin growing when a sperm leaves the man's body and joins together with an egg in the woman's body. For the sperm and egg to join, the sperm must leave the man's body through the *penis* and enter the *uterus* (or *womb*)—a special place in the woman's body where a baby can grow.

Sperm are made in a part of a man's body called the *testicles.* Sperm are very tiny, and are held in a special sac called the *scrotum,* that hangs between a boy's legs.

God has designed each boy with a **penis**, a short tube on the outside of his body, so that he can pass *urine* through it. And so that later, when he grows up and becomes a husband, his sperm can pass through it to create a baby.

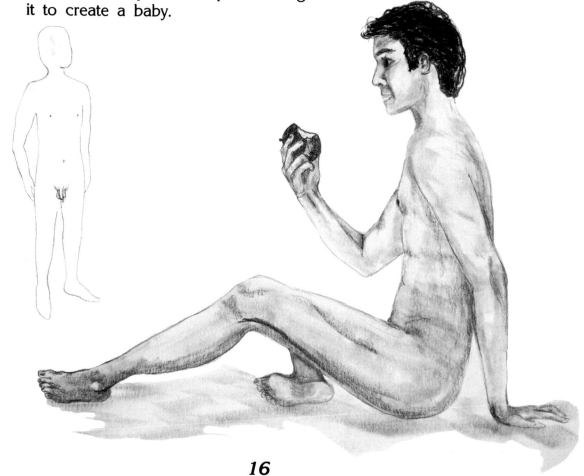

Eggs are made deep inside a woman's body in the *ovaries*. Eggs are larger than sperm but are still too small to see without using a microscope.

A woman does not have a penis. Instead, she has two separate body parts—an opening for passing urine—and another opening inside her body, for reproduction—a tube called the *vagina*. The vagina is also called the "birth canal" because a baby must pass through it to be born.

These private parts between her legs are called the *vulva*.

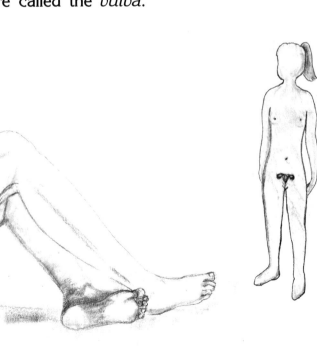

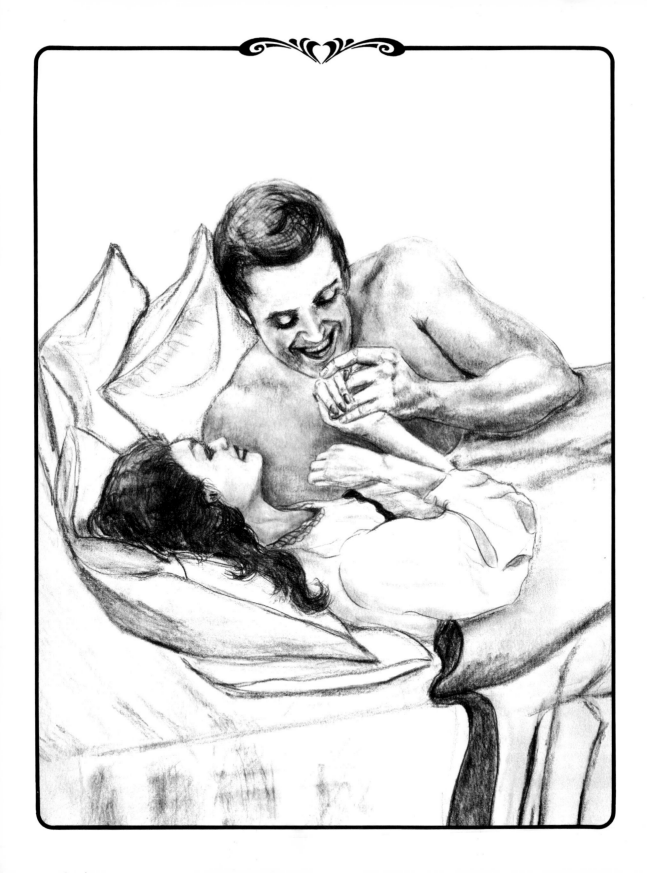

A man's body and a woman's body are made for one another. The husband's penis fits perfectly into his wife's vagina. When he places his penis inside her body we call it "sexual intercourse," "having sex," or "making love."

God's Word tells us that married couples are to make love regularly. The way people make love is private and special between the two of them. Often it involves a lot of touching, talking, and sharing. It can be lots of fun and make them happy, or it can be very serious. How often they make love depends on the couple. Husbands and wives make love when they feel very close and they both want to.

THE BEGINNING

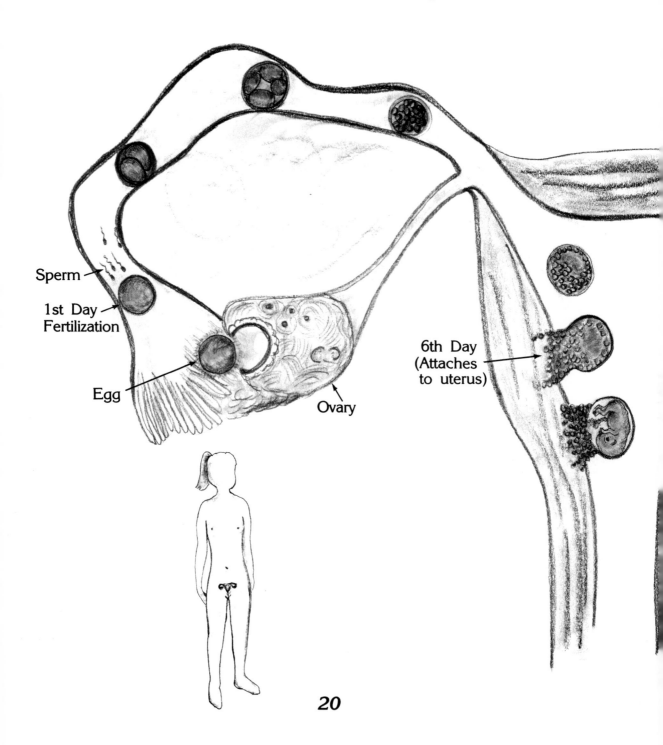

Sperm

1st Day
Fertilization

Egg

Ovary

6th Day
(Attaches
to uterus)

20

OF A NEW LIFE!

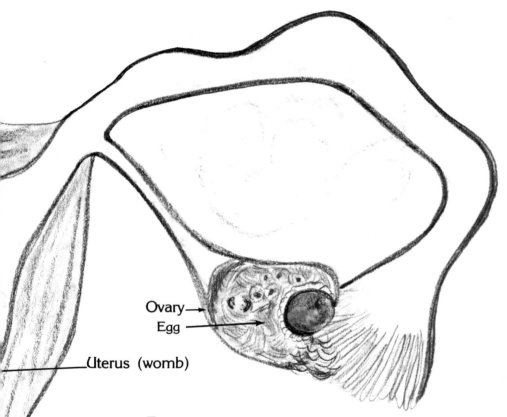

Ovary
Egg
Uterus (womb)

If an egg is released from a woman's ovary into a fallopian tube and joins with a sperm, the egg is said to be *fertilized* by the sperm. The instant this new life begins is called *conception.*

Conception doesn't always happen when people make love. People make love because it feels good and makes them happy. It helps a husband and wife feel close and loving toward one another, and reminds them they were made for each other.

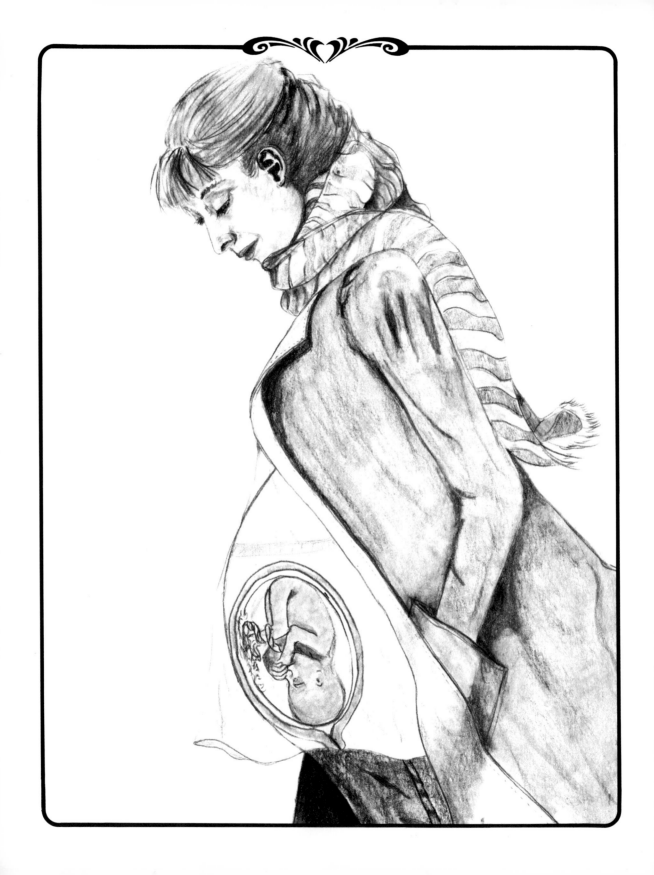

Miraculously, through God's design, the tiny fertilized egg grows, changes, and multiplies until it is a full-sized baby. It takes nine months of growing before a baby is ready to be born on its "birth day."

Some people say that a baby grows in a mommy's "tummy," but this is not exactly so. Babies grow in the uterus (womb)—that special place in a woman's body made just for protecting and feeding a new life. Inside the uterus the baby floats in a sac of fluid that cushions it from bumps and jars. The baby gets food and air from its mother through the *umbilical cord*, a soft tube that connects the mother to the middle of the baby's abdomen. After the baby is born, a "belly button" is all that is left of this cord.

A GROWING BABY IS

 At 4 weeks a new baby is only 1/4 inch long.

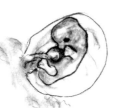 At 6 weeks brain waves can be detected.

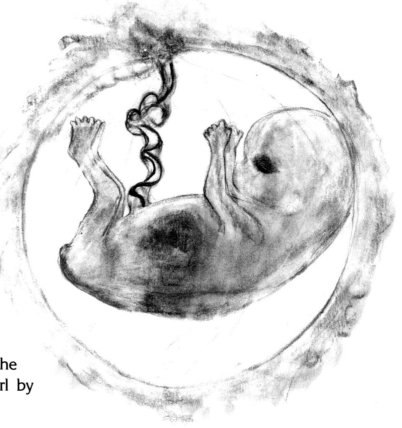

At a little over 8 weeks there are beginnings of fingers, toes, eyes, ears, a nose, and a mouth.

The heart is beating, and the baby is clearly a boy or girl by 8 weeks.

SUCH A MIRACLE OF LIFE

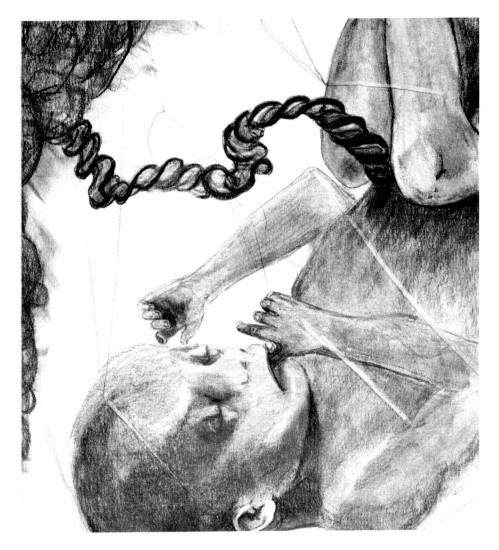

The fertilized egg from which you grew was no bigger than a grain of sand. In fourteen days your head and brain were beginning to form. Arm buds and the beginnings of eyes were visible by four weeks. At six weeks your spine could be seen, and one week later you had grown to 3/4 of an inch and were moving your hands.

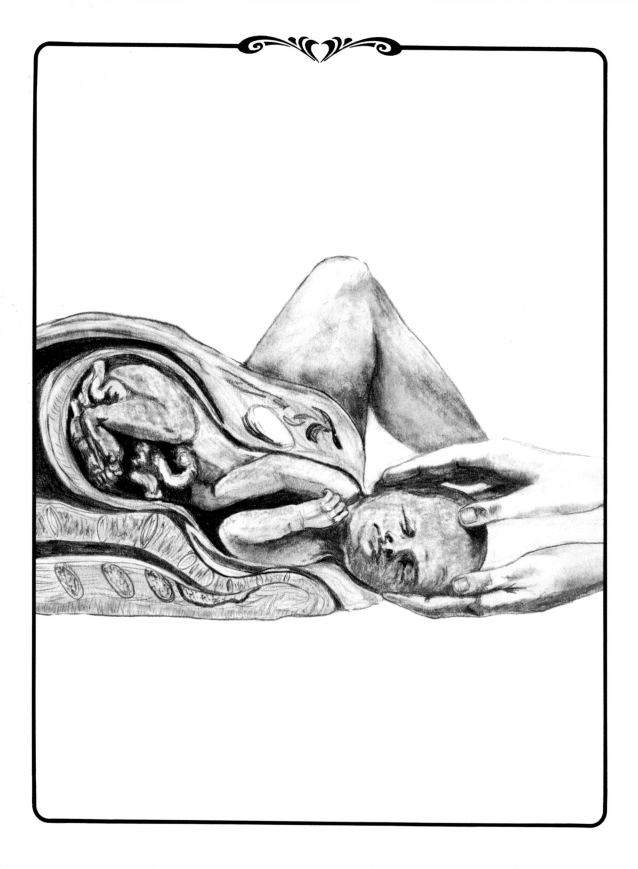

You may have heard stories about the day you were born. Because giving birth is hard work, it seems right that we call the muscle contractions of the uterus that push the baby out—*labor*. The baby moves slowly down the birth canal (vagina) and comes out the vaginal opening.

Most of the time, having a baby goes just the way it is supposed to. And because having a baby is such a special part of being a family, some people prefer to stay at home when their babies are born. But others, in case there are problems, choose to give birth in a hospital because they like to know that doctors and medicine are near to help.

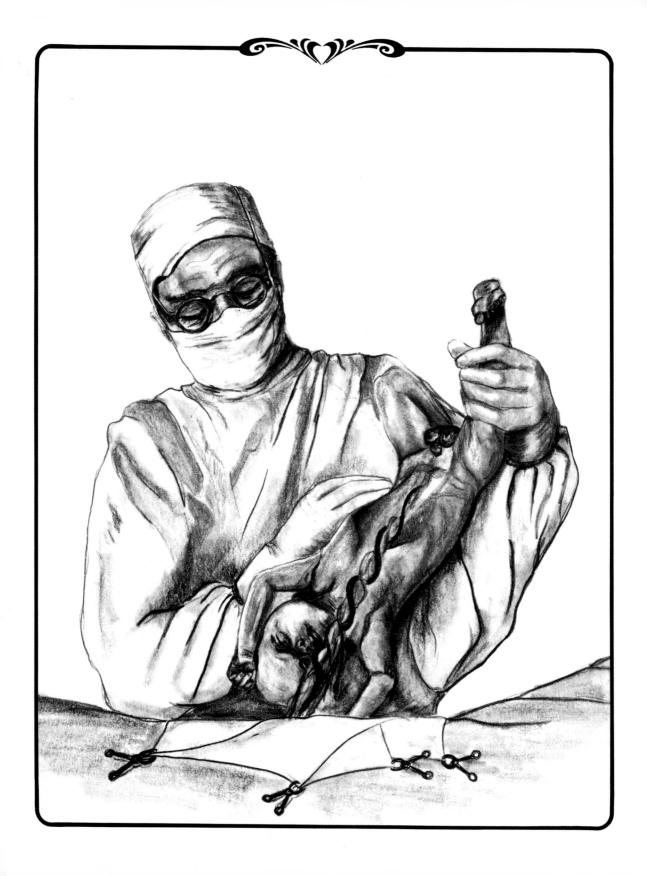

Sometimes because of a special problem, such as a baby's being very big, the baby cannot move down the birth canal. When this happens, a doctor must perform surgery. For the baby to be born, the mother is anesthetized, then the doctor makes an incision in her abdomen, and lifts the baby out. This kind of birth is called a *Caesarean* or *C-section*. Babies born by a C-section are just as healthy as those who are born the usual way.

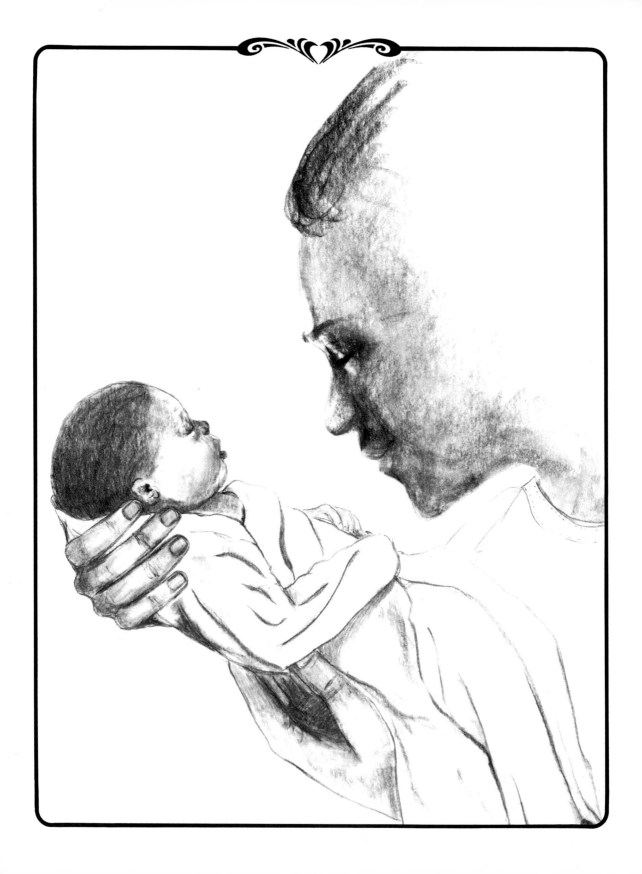

You probably don't remember the very first thing you did when you were born: It was to breathe all by yourself.

You may have heard family stories about the way you looked when you were born. Because babies, to be born, have to be pushed and squeezed through a narrow space, God designed them so that their bodies and heads will bend and stretch a little, sometimes making newborns look not very cute. And some newborns may be red, wrinkled, or have funny-shaped heads!

Before long, though, they become much better looking. Family and friends are sure their newborn is "the best looking baby in the nursery."

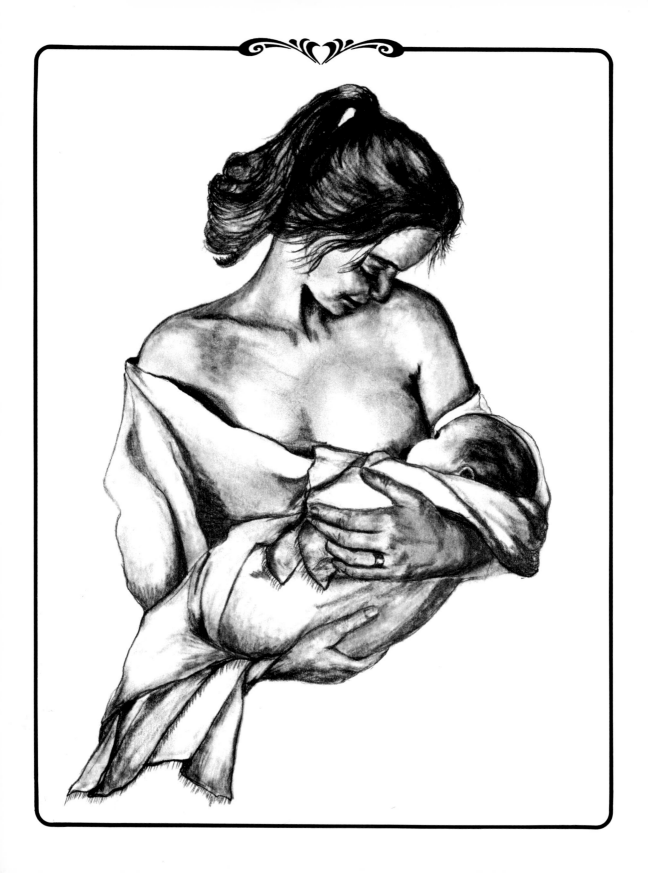

Newborns are very helpless and need everyone in the family to help take care of them. One thing they know how to do well is to suck milk from their mother's breast or from a bottle.

God gave the woman fuller breasts than the man so she could feed her baby as soon as he or she is born. A breast has a nipple right where a baby can find it when the mother holds the baby in her arms. Milk glands inside it make just the right amount of milk.

A mother's milk is the perfect food for her baby, but sometimes a mother has reasons for giving her baby milk from a bottle instead. The "formula" she buys is as close to a mother's milk as it can be. Babies will be just as healthy on either type of milk, but they MUST have lots of touching and holding.

No matter how old we are, we never outgrow our need to be touched, held—and loved.

This is why God planned for us His good gift of families.

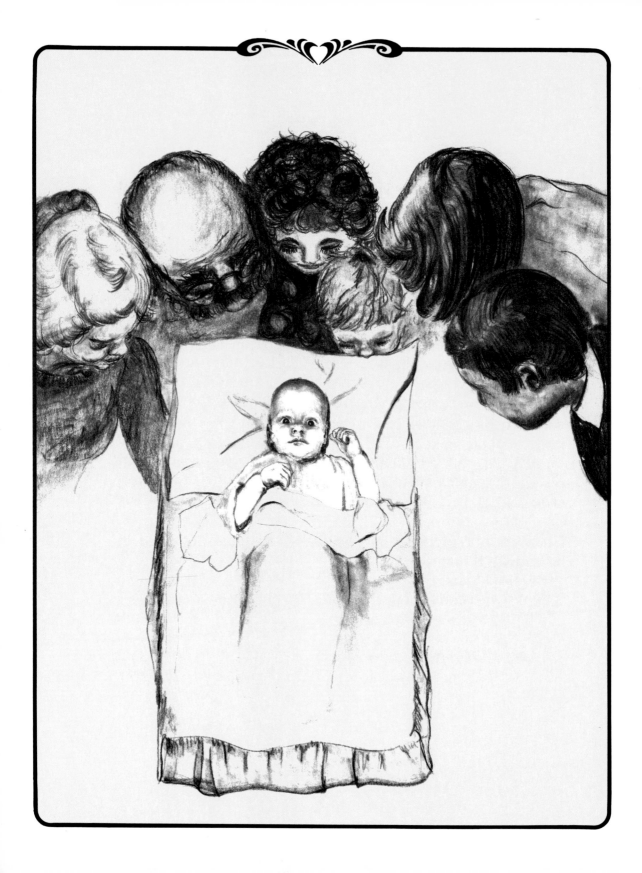

You've probably had days when you didn't think it was so great to be in a family. Maybe you wished the family next door were yours! But, good or bad, happy or sad, our own family is always special to us.

All our families could be better if we followed closely God's plan for living: **Love God with all your heart and love others the way you would like to be loved.**

God made us people who make choices. Has your mom or dad ever told you to do something, but you didn't do it? You knew what he or she wanted, but instead you did what *you* wanted to do.

Sometimes grown-ups do the very same thing. They know what God wants them to do but they decide not to listen. The temptations and distractions of the world make it hard for them to obey.

For example, a married person can become interested in people and things besides his or her family. The husband or wife may decide not to stay and be a part of the family any longer.

Others believe they know how to run their lives better than God would, and decide to live life in their way, not God's.

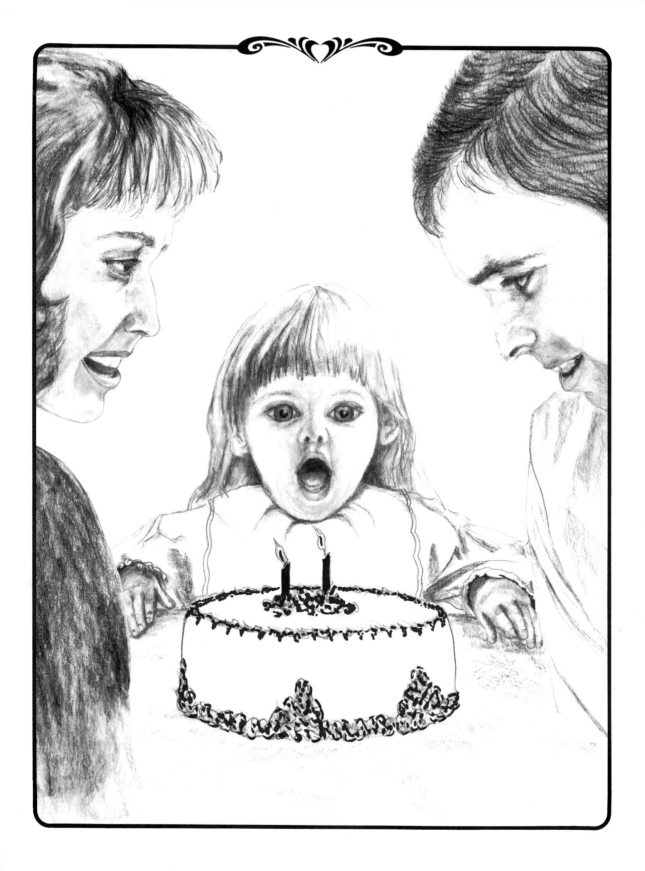

Ever wish for a perfect family? The truth is, no family is perfect. However, no matter what people do, God's plan for a woman and a man to leave their families and start a new one of their own is a great idea. Children are happiest when their mom and dad love, trust, and are committed to one another. Husbands and wives follow God's plan when they have sexual intercourse **only** with each other.

Staying faithful and committed to the family is very hard for some people ... but the peace, joy, and happiness in a family that functions the way it is supposed to, makes it worth the effort.

Families that always act loving and make kids feel safe all the time are rare. Most of us have families that try hard. We want to love each other and be the best family we can be. That is what God wants for us ... it is His plan. Some families, however, have many difficulties.

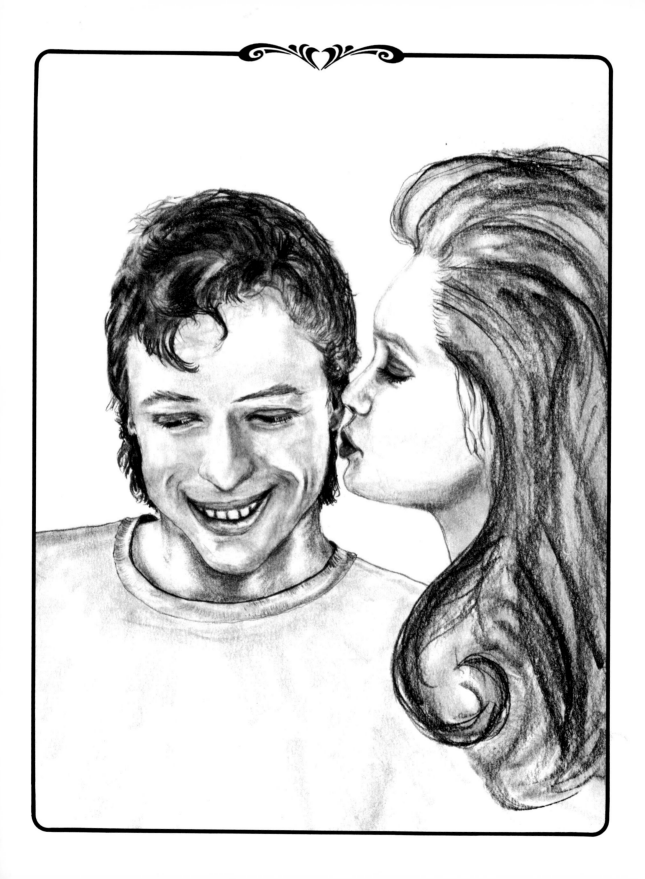

Did you know that problems in families sometimes start before the marriage? Frequently problems happen because having sexual intercourse feels good! As a matter of fact, it can be so enjoyable that some people think it's silly to limit it to one partner or to save it for marriage. Some single people decide it's just too difficult to wait.

But not waiting causes a lot of troubles. First of all, it means breaking God's rules. And that's not all—not waiting can spread diseases. God wants single people to build relationships not on sex but upon friendship, respect, and what is best for the other person.

A person who has never had sexual intercourse is called a *virgin*. An individual who has chosen not to be sexually involved with another is said to practice *abstinence*, be *abstinent*, or *celibate*.

When you get older, you will have to decide if you are going to be abstinent while you are single. God wants us to be healthy and happy. He understands what will make our lives turn out the very best. Abstinence is God's plan for people who are not married, because He knows it helps people stay healthy—physically and emotionally.

For sure, marriages are off to a good start when husbands and wives are able to promise that they will share their bodies **only** with each other. It is special to participate in lovemaking that is yours and your mate's alone.

God did not design our bodies to have sexual partners other than our own husband or wife. His plan and intent from the beginning was that families would be healthy and loving and would stay together. So when people have sex before marriage, they have decided not to follow God's plan for them. And if husbands or wives have sex with someone they are not married to, their families are hurt badly. The decision not to live by God's plan can mess up people's lives.

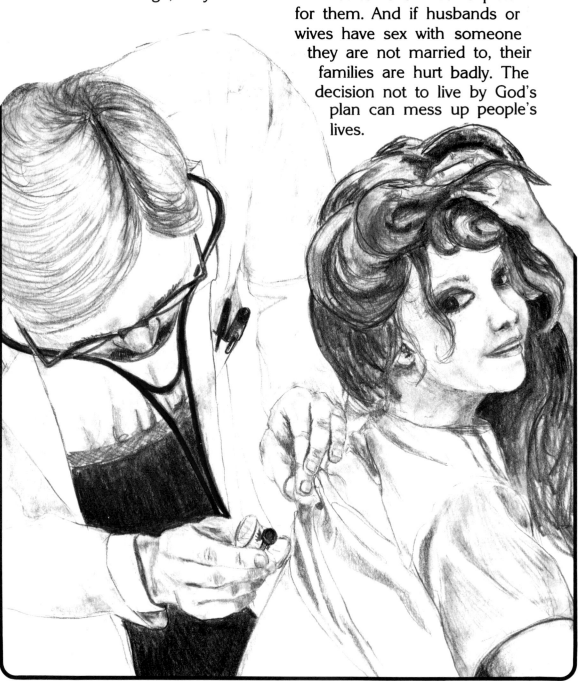

The effects on our bodies can be scary because certain diseases can be passed between people who have sex with one another. We call these *Sexually Transmitted Diseases* or *STDs* because only someone with the disease can pass it on to someone else. STDs don't float in the air as cold germs do, and are not found on objects like toilet seats. You can get the disease only if you have sexual intercourse, or some other intimate contact with an exchange of body fluids.

One STD you've probably heard a lot about is **A**cquired **I**mmune **D**eficiency **S**yndrome (AIDS). You've seen sad pictures of babies dying of AIDS, and of kids like Ryan White, who got AIDS after receiving a blood transfusion. Today, to protect those needing a transfusion, blood is tested before it is given.

It's also possible to get AIDS by using drugs illegally and sharing a needle already used by someone with AIDS. Sharing needles is a dangerous way kids or grown-ups might get AIDS and thus spread the disease. Although AIDS has been found in tears and saliva, experts tell us there's little to no chance of getting it from dishes or just being around or touching an infected person. Mostly, people get AIDS when body fluids are mixed through sex.

AIDS is frightening because there's no cure for it, and people with AIDS die much sooner than they would if they didn't have AIDS. But **you** can make choices! You can choose **not** to get involved with drugs. You can choose **not** to have sex before marriage. You can choose to marry someone who has followed God's plan just as you have.

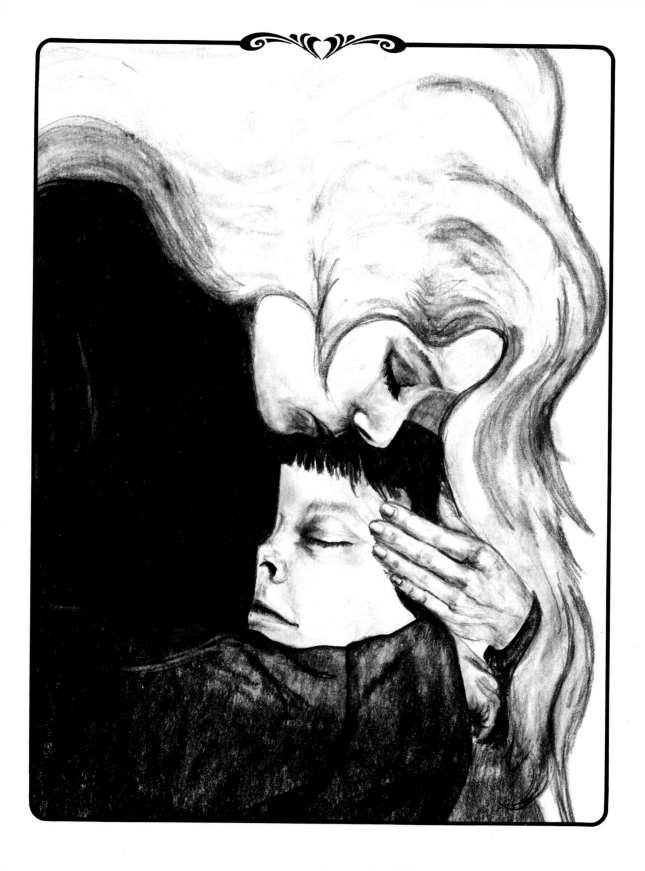

Remember when we said that sometimes people get embarrassed talking about sex? Some of those people have misunderstood and are all mixed up about what sex is supposed to be.

When a man or woman, boy or girl, doesn't understand, is too embarrassed, or can't find anyone to talk to about how to be healthy sexually, then life doesn't work out as it should. Sometimes people who misunderstand their sexuality may force a child to touch their private parts, or they may touch a child's private parts They may even have sexual intercourse. This is called "molestation" or "sexual abuse."

Everyone likes and needs to be touched, and kids don't have to worry that hugs and cuddles in the right way by people they know and trust are wrong. But children need to know that **no one** has a right to touch their bodies in a way that makes them feel uncomfortable. Even if a child likes the attention and the feelings—molestation is wrong. So no matter how polite you usually are, it **is** all right to say NO!

A child who has been molested should never worry that God is angry at him or her, or that being molested was his or her fault. It's tough for some molested kids to feel good about themselves because they are sure they must have done something wrong for such a thing to have happened to them. They feel ashamed. What has happened to them is sad and bad, but they need to be reminded they are still the beautiful kids God planned for ... before they were even born.

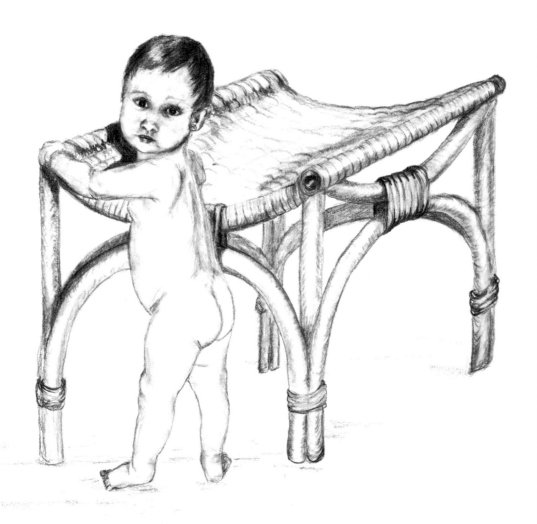

Most likely in your family album there is a picture of you as a baby in your "birthday suit." You are probably smiling out at the world as happily as can be! Whenever your family looks through the album or shows it to friends, you may get lovingly teased about your baby picture. We know for sure it was taken by proud parents who thought you had the most adorable, sweetest little body of any baby ever!

But there are pictures of children and grown-ups that aren't cute. They are taken for people who don't know how to follow God's plan for us to enjoy sex. We call such material *pornography.* In the past, many people thought that looking at sexy pictures and movies didn't hurt much. Today we know they can do a lot of harm.

Pornography hurts women because it makes its viewers think of women not as mothers, workers, and interesting people but as persons just to have sex with. It hurts children, too, because it teaches things about sex that are not true.

Pornography declares that it's okay to have sex without a loving relationship. Sometimes it suggests that sex and violence go together. **Nothing could be further from the truth.**

The sex act is meant to be a *caring* act that has nothing to do with hurting or mistreating anyone. Sex is to have meaning because of the relationship between a husband and his wife. It was designed as a special way grown-ups who love one another have of being close.

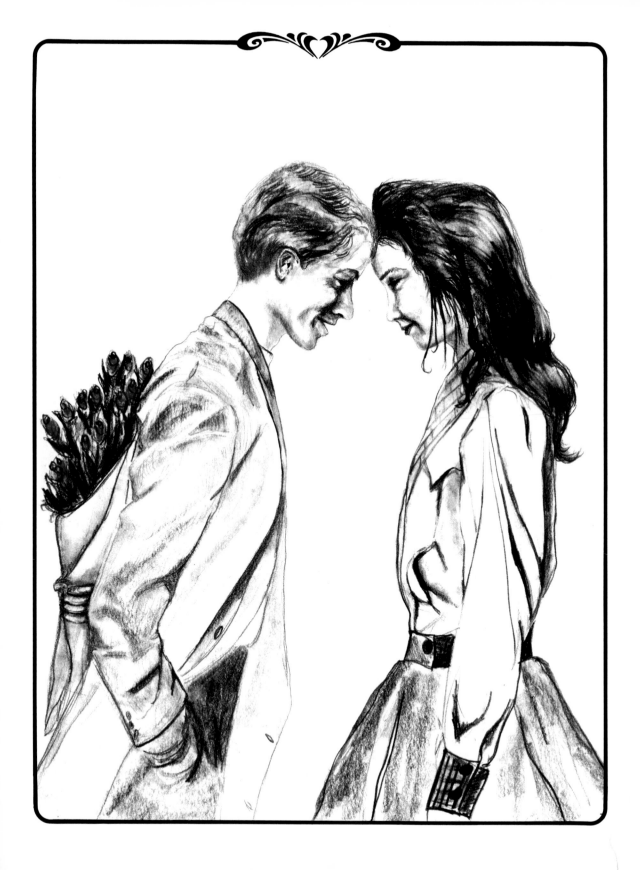

Isn't it great that God decided to make two sexes? (He didn't have to—He could have made us like the one-cell amoeba that just divides into two new pieces.) Since God did make us people who make choices, He expects us to make good choices about how we treat our bodies.

How do you know you will make good choices?—because you have been told the **truth:** *Sexual intercourse is designed for a permanent relationship in marriage—to be between husbands and wives.* When individuals decide to have sex with persons they are not married to anyway, many sad things can happen—pregnancies, abortions, diseases, and unhappy and difficult relationships. Many people say that making the wrong decisions about sexuality has been the worst mistake of their lives.

Even though it seems that most people ignore the truth, it is important for you to remember that God's plan is not the problem. His plan is sometimes hard to follow because some people, some movies, some records, and our own feelings tell us not to wait until we are married to have sex.

When pressures are too great ... you need God's help. Make sure you hang around with kids who also know the truth. Go to your mom and dad with any questions you have about sex. If they are embarrassed, try your youth pastor, a teacher, a nurse, or a doctor.

God's design of two sexes is **good**. It was not intended to be a mystery or source of pain. Make sure that in your life, the *gift* of sex is all God meant it to be!